WEIGHT GAI COOKBOOK FUR BEGINNERS

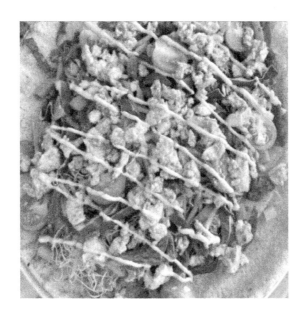

Easy and Friendly High Calorie Recipes For Healthy Weight Gain And Body Building

THERESA EATON

Copyright ©2023 by Theresa Eaton

This book is intended to provide helpful and informative material on the subject matter covered. Every effort has been made to ensure that the information in this book is accurate and up-to-date at the time of the publication. However the author does not warrant that the information contained therein is complete or free from error.

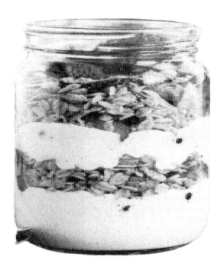

Table of Contents

INTRODUCTION

While many people concentrate on losing weight, some people have trouble with the opposite problem: gaining weight. This book is here to support you on your journey, whether you have a naturally quick metabolism, a busy lifestyle, or particular medical conditions that make it difficult for you to gain weight.

The first step is realizing the significance of weight gain. Many people might mistakenly think that gaining weight can be accomplished by simply eating more junk food or making bad decisions. However, developing a balanced diet that encourages muscle growth, boosts energy levels, and supports general well-being is the key to effective and long-lasting weight gain.

We will examine the basic ideas behind weight gain in this book, along with the variables that influence it and goal-setting techniques.

This book's extensive collection of recipes is what makes it so special. Every chapter focuses on a different meal, such as breakfast, lunch, dinner, snacks, or even dessert. These recipes have been carefully chosen to offer you a wide selection of delicious, quick, and calorie-rich options that are high in nutrients. You'll find a wide variety of options to suit your taste buds and dietary preferences, ranging from breakfasts packed with protein to filling dinners and decadent desserts.

In addition to the recipes, we'll give you useful advice so you can succeed in your weight-gain endeavours. We'll look at how to monitor your development, make necessary dietary changes, incorporate exercise and strength training, and get past typical roadblocks. We will provide you with the resources you need to maintain your motivation and consistency while achieving your weight gain objectives.

Keep in mind that gaining weight healthily and sustainably takes time, commitment, and a well-rounded strategy. This book is here to help you every step of the way, providing insightful information, delectable recipes, and professional guidance to support you on your journey to a healthier and more balanced body.

Let's set out on this journey together, and along the way, let the "Weight Gain Diet Cookbook For Beginners" be your dependable travel companion.

CHAPTER 1

Understanding Weight Gain and Its Importance

Weight gain is the term used to describe an increase in body weight, which typically happens when there is an imbalance between energy intake (calories consumed) and energy expenditure (calories burned). Gaining weight can have a big impact on one's general health and well-being, so it's important to understand it. The risk of developing various diseases, including heart disease, diabetes, some cancers, and musculoskeletal disorders, is lower when one maintains a healthy weight. Gaining weight can also have an impact on one's quality of life, self-esteem, and body image.

Why Does Weight Gain Matter?

Gaining weight is important because it can cause obesity, which is a major health concern in the world if it is excessive or uncontrolled. Obesity has been linked to an increased risk of chronic illnesses like respiratory problems, type 2 diabetes, cancer, and cardiovascular disease.

Furthermore, it may shorten life expectancy and aggravate mental health problems. Individuals can make wise decisions to manage their weight and enhance their health outcomes by having a thorough understanding of weight gain and its effects.

Factors Affecting Weight Gain

Many variables can affect weight gain, including:

1. **Intake of Calories:** Consuming more calories than your body requires can result in weight gain. Consuming too many calories can be caused by high-calorie foods that are high in fats and sugars.

2. **Exercise:** A sedentary lifestyle with little exercise can lower energy expenditure and cause weight gain. Calorie burn and maintaining a healthy weight are both helped by regular exercise.

3. **Genetics:** An individual's propensity to gain weight may be influenced by genetic factors. A higher genetic propensity to store extra weight may exist in some individuals.

4. **Factors relating to hormones:** Weight gain can be influenced by hormonal imbalances like hypothyroidism and polycystic ovary syndrome (PCOS), which affect metabolism.

5. **Medications:** Antidepressants, antipsychotics, and corticosteroids are a few examples of drugs that can have the side effect of weight gain.

6. **Emotional Factor:** The use of food as a coping mechanism for stress, anxiety, or other emotions, such as emotional eating, can result in weight gain.

Setting Achievable Goals

Setting attainable goals is crucial for managing weight. To help you set realistic goals, consider the following advice:

1. **Seek advice from a medical expert:** Speak with a registered dietitian or medical expert who can evaluate your health, make individualized recommendations, and assist you in establishing reasonable weight goals.

2. **Pay attention to overall well-being:** Don't just pay attention to the number on the scale; also think about enhancing your overall well-being by improving your diet and getting more exercise. Maintain a balanced, healthy lifestyle as your goal.

3. **Set clear, attainable goals:** Establish clear objectives like losing a certain amount of weight or measuring less than a certain amount of inches over a certain time frame. For the sake of racking your progress, make sure your goals are measurable.

4. **Make Gradual Changes:** Avoid drastic or unsustainable dietary or exercise regimen changes by making them gradually. Make gradual, small changes to establish long-lasting routines instead.

5. **Have patience and perseverance:** Healthy weight loss or gain requires time. Keep focused on your goals and try not to let slow progress demotivate you.

As you should always keep in mind, achieving your ideal weight should not come before your general health and well-being.

CHAPTER 2

BREAKFAST RECIPES

High-Calorie Smoothie Bowl

Servings: 1

Cooking time: 10 minutes

Ingredients:

- 1 cup whole milk or plant-based milk
- 1 large banana
- Two teaspoons of nut butter, such as peanut or almond butter
- 1/4 cup rolled oats
- 1 tablespoon honey or maple syrup
- 1 tablespoon chia seeds
- 1 tablespoon ground flaxseed
- Your preferred toppings, such as granola, nuts, or coconut flakes, may be used.

Instructions:

1. Blend the milk, banana, nut butter, rolled oats, honey or maple syrup, chia seeds, and ground flaxseed in a food processor or blender.

2. Blend till it becomes creamy and smooth.

3. Carry a bowl and transfer the mixture inside.

4. Add your preferred garnishes, such as granola, nuts, coconut flakes, and sliced fruit.

5. Savour the calorie-dense smoothie bowl!

Protein Pancakes with Toppings

Servings: 2

Cooking time: 20 minutes

Ingredients:

- 1 cup all-purpose flour
- 1 scoop protein powder (your preferred flavour)
- 1 tablespoon sugar
- 1 teaspoon baking powder
- 1/2 teaspoon baking soda
- 1/4 teaspoon salt
- 1 cup buttermilk or milk of your choice
- 1 large egg
- 2 tablespoons melted butter or oil
- Toppings of your choice (e.g., sliced fruits, nuts, yoghurt, syrup)

Instructions:

1. Mix the flour, protein powder, sugar, baking soda, salt, and baking powder and whisk them in a big bowl.

2. Whisk the buttermilk, egg, and melted butter or oil in a different bowl.

3. After adding the wet ingredients, stir the dry ingredients only until they are barely combined. Avoid over mixing; the batter should still have some lumps.

4. Over medium temperature, preheat a nonstick skillet or griddle.

5. For each pancake, pour 1/4 cup of batter into the skillet.

6. Cook till surface bubbles appear, then turn to the other side and continue to cook until golden brown.

7. Continue the process by using the remaining batter.

8. Dish the protein pancakes alongside your preferred toppings, such as yoghurt, syrup, sliced fruit, nuts, and nuts.

Avocado and Egg Toast

Servings: 1

Cooking time: 10 minutes

Ingredients:

- 1 slice of bread (whole grain or your preference), toasted
- 1 ripe avocado
- 1 large egg
- Salt and pepper to taste
- Optional toppings: Cut-up tomatoes, feta cheese, red pepper flakes

Instructions:

1. Remove the avocado's pit, then cut it in half. Scoop the flesh into a small container.

2. Use a fork to mash the avocado to the consistency you want.

3. Season the mashed avocado by sprinkling it with salt and pepper to taste.

4. Cook the egg in a nonstick skillet however you like it (fried, scrambled, poached, etc.).

5. On the toasted bread, evenly distribute the mashed avocado.

6. Over the avocado, place the scrambled egg.

7. You can also choose to add extras like feta cheese, sliced tomatoes, or red pepper flakes.

8. Put more salt and pepper to taste, if you like.

9. Enjoy the toast with avocado and eggs!

Oatmeal Power Bowl

Servings: 1

Cooking time: 10 minutes

Ingredients:
- 1/2 cup rolled oats
- 1 cup whole milk or plant-based milk
- One teaspoon of nut butter, such as almond or peanut butter
- 1 tablespoon honey or maple syrup
- 1 tablespoon chia seeds
- 1 tablespoon ground flaxseed
- Toppings of your choice (e.g., sliced fruits, nuts, seeds, cinnamon)

Instructions:

1. Milk and rolled oats should be added in a small saucepan.

2. Cook the oats for between five and seven minutes over medium heat, stirring occasionally, until they are soft and the mixture has thickened.

3. Add the nut butter, honey or maple syrup, chia seeds, and ground flaxseed after taking the pan off the heat.

4. Oatmeal should be transferred to a bowl.

5. Add any extras you like, like chopped nuts, seeds, or cinnamon.

6. Enjoy your oatmeal power bowl after mixing everything!

Energy-Packed Breakfast Burrito

Servings: 2

Cooking time: 20 minutes

Ingredients:

- 4 large eggs
- 1 tablespoon olive oil
- 1/4 cup diced onions
- 1/4 cup diced bell peppers
- 1/4 cup diced tomatoes
- 1/4 cup shredded cheese (your preferred type)
- 2 large tortillas (whole wheat or flour)
- Salt and pepper to taste
- Optional fillings: cooked bacon, sausage, avocado, spinach, etc.

Instructions:

1. Whisk the eggs in a bowl and add pepper and salt to taste.

2. Over medium temperature, warm up the olive oil in a skillet.

3. Pour and cook the tomatoes, bell peppers, and diced onions in the skillet until they are soft.

4. In the skillet with the cooked vegetables, add the beaten eggs and scramble them until they are fully cooked.

5. Over the scrambled eggs, scatter the cheese crumbles, and stir until it melts.

6. Use a microwave or a different skillet to reheat the tortillas.

7. Between the tortillas, divide the egg and cheese mixture.

8. You can also choose to add extra ingredients like cooked bacon, sausage, avocado, or spinach.

9. Create burritos by rolling the tortillas.

10. The energizing breakfast burritos should be served warm.

Banana Nut Overnight Oats

Servings: 1

Preparation time: 5 minutes (plus overnight chilling)

Ingredients:

- 1/2 cup rolled oats
- 1/2 cup milk of your choice
- 1 ripe banana, mashed
- One teaspoon of nut butter, such as almond or peanut butter
- 1 tablespoon honey or maple syrup
- 1 tablespoon chopped nuts (e.g., walnuts, almonds, pecans)
- Optional toppings: sliced banana, additional chopped nuts, a drizzle of honey

Instructions:

1. Rolled oats, milk, mashed banana, nut butter, and honey or maple syrup should all be added to a jar or other container.

2. Make sure to thoroughly mix all the ingredients by giving them a good stir.

3. Place the container or jar in the refrigerator covered for at least four hours or overnight.

4. Give the overnight oats a good mix in the morning.

5. Add chopped nuts and any additional toppings, like sliced banana and honey, to taste.

6. Enjoy your wholesome overnight oats with bananas and nuts!

Veggie Breakfast Scramble

Servings: 2

Cooking time: 15 minutes

Ingredients:
- 4 large eggs
- 1 tablespoon olive oil
- 1/4 cup diced onions
- 1/4 cup diced bell peppers
- 1/4 cup diced zucchini
- 1/4 cup diced mushrooms
- Salt and pepper to taste
- Optional toppings: shredded cheese, chopped fresh herbs (e.g., parsley, chives)

Instructions:

1. Over a medium flame, warm up the olive oil in a skillet.

2. In the skillet, add the diced onions, bell peppers, zucchini, and mushrooms. Vegetables should be simmered till they are tender.

3. Salt and pepper the eggs in a bowl after whisking them.

4. Pour the beaten eggs into the other side of the skillet while pushing the cooked vegetables to one side.

5. The eggs should be scrambled and cooked till they are no more runny.

6. The scrambled eggs should be combined with the cooked vegetables.

7. Add optional toppings like shredded cheese and finely chopped fresh herbs after removing from the heat.

8. Enjoy the warm veggie breakfast scramble by serving it!

Sweet Potato Hash with Eggs

Servings: 2

Cooking time: 25 minutes

Ingredients:

- 2 medium sweet potatoes, peeled and cubed
- 1 tablespoon olive oil
- 1/2 cup diced onions
- 1/2 cup diced bell peppers
- 2 cloves garlic, minced
- 1 teaspoon paprika
- 1/2 teaspoon cumin
- Salt and pepper to taste
- 4 large eggs
- Optional toppings: chopped fresh herbs (e.g., parsley, cilantro), hot sauce

Instructions:

1. Olive oil should be heated in a sizable skillet over a medium flame.

2. Stirring now and then, add the sweet potatoes and cook until they begin to soften.

3. In the skillet, add the diced onions, bell peppers, and garlic.

4. Cook the vegetables and sweet potatoes further in the same manner until they are both soft.

5. Cumin and paprika should be added to the sweet potato mixture.

6. To taste, add salt and pepper to the food. The spices should be thoroughly mixed into the vegetables.

7. Four holes should be made in the sweet potato hash, and each one should contain a cracked egg in it.

8. Cook the eggs in a covered skillet for about five to seven minutes, or until they are cooked to your preference.

9. Remove from heat and top with optional garnishes like hot sauce and finely chopped fresh herbs.

10. Enjoy the hot sweet potato hash with eggs!

Chia Pudding with Berries

Servings: 2

Preparation time: 5 minutes (plus chilling time)

Ingredients:

- 1/4 cup chia seeds
- 1 cup milk of your choice (e.g., almond milk, coconut milk)
- 1 tablespoon honey or maple syrup
- 1/2 teaspoon vanilla extract
- 1 cup mixed berries (e.g., strawberries, blueberries, blackberries)
- Optional toppings: sliced almonds, shredded coconut, a drizzle of honey

Instructions:

1. Chia seeds, milk, honey or maple syrup, and vanilla extract should all be added to a bowl.

2. To prevent the chia seeds from clumping together, thoroughly stir the mixture to distribute them evenly.

3. Once the chia seeds have absorbed the liquid and taken on the consistency of pudding, cover the bowl and place it in the refrigerator for at least two hours (or overnight).

4. Before serving, stir the chia pudding to break up any clumps.

5. Put the chia pudding into two bowls or glasses for serving.

6. Add mixed berries and any additional toppings, such as honey drizzles, shredded coconut, or almond slices, to each serving.

7. Take pleasure in the delicious and healthy chia pudding with berries!

High-Calorie Oatmeal

Servings: 1

Cooking Time: 10 minutes

Ingredients:

- 1/2 cup rolled oats
- 1 cup whole milk
- 2 tablespoons nut butter (e.g., almond or peanut butter)
- 1 tablespoon honey or maple syrup
- A quarter cup of chopped nuts, such as almonds, walnuts, or cashews
- 1/4 cup dried fruits (e.g., raisins, cranberries, or apricots)

Instructions:

1. The whole milk and rolled oats should be added to a saucepan.

2. Cook the oats till the mixture becomes thickened for approximately five to seven minutes on a medium flame, stirring occasionally.

3. Then turn off the heat and thoroughly combine the nut butter, honey, and maple syrup in the saucepan.

4. Put the oatmeal in a bowl for serving.

5. Add chopped nuts and dried fruit on top.

CHAPTER 3

LUNCH RECIPES

Creamy Chicken Pasta

Servings: 2

Cooking Time: 30 minutes

Ingredients:

- 8 ounces of boneless, skinless chicken breasts
- 6 ounces of whole-wheat pasta
- 1 tablespoon of olive oil
- 1 cup of heavy cream
- 1 cup of grated Parmesan cheese
- 1 cup of broccoli florets
- Salt and pepper to taste

Instructions:

1. As directed on the packaging, cook the pasta. Drain, then set apart.

2. In a pan, warm up the olive oil over medium flame.

3. The chicken breasts should be salt and pepper-seasoned, and they should be cooked through and browned in the pan.

4. Move the Chicken from the pan and set it to one side.

5. Put the heavy cream and Parmesan cheese in the same pan.

6. Stir continuously until the sauce thickens and the cheese melts.

7. Combine the sauce with the cooked pasta and broccoli florets.

8. Stir everything until it is completely coated.

9. Add the sliced cooked chicken to the pasta.

10. Cook for a further two to three minutes, or until thoroughly heated.

11. Serve and savour while hot.

Beef and Vegetable Stir-Fry

Servings: 4

Cooking Time: 20 minutes

Ingredients:

- 1 pound of beef sirloin, thinly sliced
- Two cups of mixed vegetables, such as carrots, bell peppers, and broccoli
- 2 tablespoons of soy sauce
- 1 tablespoon of cornstarch
- 1 tablespoon of vegetable oil
- 2 cloves of garlic, minced
- Salt and pepper to taste

Instructions:

1. Combine the soy sauce, cornstarch, salt, and pepper in a small bowl and whisk, then Place aside.

2. In a big skillet or wok, warm up the vegetable oil over high heat.

3. Stir-fry the minced garlic for about thirty seconds after adding it.

5. Stir-fry the beef slices in the skillet until they are well-browned and cooked.

6. Stir-fry the mixed vegetables in the skillet for an additional two to three minutes, or until crisp-tender.

7. Transfer the soy sauce mixture over the beef and vegetables. Once everything is thoroughly covered, cook for one more minute to allow the sauce to thicken.

8. Serve hot with rice or noodles after removing from the heat.

Loaded Sweet Potato

Servings: 2

Cooking Time: 1 hour

Ingredients:
- 2 large sweet potatoes
- One cup of cleaned and drained black beans
- 1 avocado, sliced
- ½ cup of shredded cheddar cheese
- ¼ cup of Greek yoghurt
- 2 green onions, sliced
- Salt and pepper to taste

Instructions:

1. Set the oven's temperature to 400°F (200°C).

2. After washing, poke the sweet potatoes several times with a fork.

3. They should be baked for forty-five to sixty minutes, or until tender, on a baking sheet.

4. The Sweet potatoes should be taken out of the oven and given some time to cool down.

5. Divide each potato lengthwise.

6. Place black beans, avocado slices, grated cheddar cheese, Greek yoghurt, and green onions inside each sweet potato.

7. To get a taste, season the food with salt and pepper.

8. Enjoy the stuffed sweet potatoes while they're hot.

Chickpea and Spinach Curry

Servings: 4

Cooking Time:25 minutes

Ingredients:

- 2 tablespoons of vegetable oil
- 1 onion, finely chopped
- 3 cloves of garlic, minced
- 1 tablespoon of curry powder
- 1 teaspoon of ground cumin
- 1 teaspoon of ground coriander
- ½ teaspoon of turmeric
- 1 can (14 ounces) of chickpeas, drained and rinsed
- 1 can (14 ounces) of diced tomatoes
- 2 cups of fresh spinach leaves
- Salt and pepper to taste
- Cooked rice or naan bread for serving

Instructions:

1. In a sizable skillet or saucepan set over medium flame, warm up the vegetable oil.

2. Add the minced garlic and onion, and cook till the onion is translucent and soft.

3. Turmeric, ground cumin, ground coriander, and curry powder should all be added to the pan.

4. Cook the onion and garlic for another minute after thoroughly mixing in the spices.

5. To the pan, add the diced tomatoes and chickpeas.

6. After stirring to combine everything, turn the heat down and simmer for ten to fifteen seconds to let the flavours meld.

7. When the spinach has begun to wilt, add the spinach leaves to the pan and cook for an additional two to three minutes.

8. To get a taste, season the food with salt and pepper.

9. Curry made with chickpeas and spinach should be served with naan bread or overcooked rice.

Tuna and Avocado Wrap

Servings: 2

Preparation Time: 10 minutes

Ingredients:

- 1 can (5 ounces) of tuna, drained
- 1 ripe avocado, mashed
- 2 large whole wheat tortillas
- ½ cup of shredded lettuce
- ½ cup of diced tomatoes
- 2 tablespoons of mayonnaise
- Salt and pepper to taste

Instructions:

1. The drained tuna, mashed avocado, mayonnaise, salt, and pepper should all be combined in a bowl.

2. The tuna and avocado filling should be well combined.

3. On a level surface, spread out the whole wheat tortillas. On each tortilla, evenly distribute the tuna and avocado filling.

4. Add diced tomatoes and lettuce on top of the filling.

5. The tortillas should be tightly rolled, with the sides folded in as you go.

6. Serve each wrap by cutting it in half.

Loaded Turkey Wrap

Servings: 2

Preparation Time: 15 minutes

Ingredients:

- 4 large whole wheat tortillas
- 8 slices of turkey breast
- 1/2 cup of hummus
- 1/2 cup of shredded cheddar cheese
- 1/2 cup of sliced cucumbers
- 1/2 cup of shredded carrots
- 1/4 cup of diced red onions
- Salt and pepper to taste

Instructions:
1. On a neat and clean surface, spread out the whole wheat tortillas.

2. On each tortilla, evenly distribute two tablespoons of hummus.

3. Each tortilla should have 2 slices of turkey breast on it.

4. Over the turkey, distribute shredded cheddar cheese, cucumber slices, carrot shreds, and red onion dice.

5. To get a taste, season the food with salt and pepper.

6. The tortillas should be firmly rolled, with the sides folded in as you go.

7. Serve the wraps by cutting them in half.

Cheesy Baked Potatoes

Servings: 4

Cooking Time: 1 hour 15 minutes

Ingredients:

- 4 large baking potatoes
- 1 cup of shredded cheddar cheese
- 1/2 cup of sour cream
- 4 tablespoons of butter

- 4 slices of cooked bacon, crumbled
- Salt and pepper to taste
- Chopped chives for garnish (optional)

Instructions:

1. Set the oven's temperature to 400°F (200°C).

2. Cleanse the baking potatoes by scrubbing them before forking them several times.

3. When the potatoes are tender when poked with a fork, place them directly on the oven rack and bake for 60 to 75 minutes.

4. The potatoes should be taken out of the oven and given some time to cool.

5. Slice each potato lengthwise, then use a fork to fluff the interiors.

6. Each potato should have butter, sour cream, bacon bits, and cheddar cheese sprinkled on top.

7. To get a taste, season the food with salt and pepper.

8. Once the cheese is melted and bubbling, return the potatoes to the oven for an additional 5 to 10 minutes.

9. If desired, garnish with finely chopped chives before serving.

Protein-Packed Lentil Salad

Servings: 4

Cooking Time: 30 minutes

Ingredients:

- 1 cup of green lentils
- 2 cups of water
- 1/2 cup of diced red bell pepper
- 1/2 cup of diced cucumber
- 1/4 cup of diced red onions
- 1/4 cup of chopped fresh parsley
- 2 tablespoons of olive oil
- 2 tablespoons of lemon juice
- 1 teaspoon of Dijon mustard
- Salt and pepper to taste

Instructions:

1. Put the green lentils in cold water and rinse.

2. The lentils and water should be combined in a saucepan.

3. Bring the lentils to a boil, then lower the heat and simmer for 20 to 25 minutes.

4. Cooked lentils should be drained and allowed to slightly cool.

5. Combine the cooked lentils with the diced red bell pepper, cucumber, red onion, and fresh parsley in a big bowl.

6. Mix the olive oil, lemon juice, Dijon mustard, salt, and pepper in a small bowl.

7. The lentil mixture should be drizzled with the dressing, then gently mixed.

8. Before serving, let the salad sit in the marinade for at least 10 minutes to let the flavours meld.

9. The lentil salad can be served cold or at room temperature.

Salmon and Quinoa Salad

Servings: 2

Preparation Time: 20 minutes

Ingredients:

- 2 salmon fillets
- 1 cup of cooked quinoa
- 2 cups of mixed salad greens
- 1/2 cucumber, sliced
- 1/4 cup of cherry tomatoes, halved
- 1/4 cup of sliced red onions
- 2 tablespoons of lemon juice
- 2 tablespoons of olive oil
- Salt and pepper to taste

Instructions:

1. Set the oven's temperature to 400°F (200°C).

2. Give the salmon fillets some salt and pepper.

3. On a baking sheet covered with parchment paper, arrange them.

4. Bake the salmon for twelve to fifteen minutes till it becomes cooked through and flakes quickly with a fork.

5. The cooked quinoa, mixed salad greens, cucumber slices, cherry tomatoes, and thinly sliced red onions should all be combined in a big bowl.

6. Lemon juice, olive oil, salt, and pepper should all be combined in a small mixing container to make the dressing.

7. As you pour the dressing over the salad, toss it to evenly distribute it.

8. Place a baked salmon fillet on top of each plate after dividing the salad among them.

9. Serve right away.

Loaded Chicken Salad Sandwich

Servings: 2

Preparation Time: 15 minutes

Ingredients:

- 2 cups of cooked chicken, shredded
- 1/2 cup of mayonnaise
- 1/4 cup of diced celery
- 1/4 cup of diced red onions
- 1/4 cup of dried cranberries

- 1/4 cup of chopped pecans
- Salt and pepper to taste
- 4 slices of whole-grain bread
- Lettuce leaves and sliced tomatoes for serving

Instructions:

1. Shredded chicken, mayonnaise, diced celery, diced red onions, dried cranberries, chopped pecans, salt, and pepper should all be combined in a bowl. Blend thoroughly.

2. If you like, toast the slices of whole-grain bread.

3. Onto two slices of bread, spread the chicken salad evenly.

4. Add lettuce and thinly sliced tomatoes to the top of each.

5. To make the remaining sandwiches, add the remaining bread slices on top.

6. If desired, cut the sandwiches in half before serving.

CHAPTER 4

DINNER RECIPES

Creamy Chicken Alfredo

Servings: 4

Cooking time: 30 minutes

Ingredients:

- 12 ounces of fettuccine pasta
- 2 tablespoons butter
- 1 pound chicken breast, sliced
- 2 cloves garlic, minced
- 1 cup heavy cream
- 1 cup grated Parmesan cheese
- Salt and pepper to taste

Instructions:

1. To prepare the fettuccine pasta, follow the directions on the package. Drain, then set apart.

2. Melt the butter in a sizable skillet over a medium flame.

4. Pour the garlic on the chicken and continue cooking till it's no longer pink.

5. Add the heavy cream, then simmer the mixture.

6. As the sauce thickens, add the Parmesan cheese and stir until it melts.

7. To get a taste, season the food with salt and pepper.

8. Pasta that has been cooked should be thoroughly coated in sauce.

9. Enjoy and serve while hot.

Beef and Broccoli Stir-Fry

Servings: 4

Cooking time: 20 minutes

Ingredients:
- 1 pound beef sirloin, thinly sliced
- 3 cups broccoli florets
- 2 tablespoons vegetable oil
- 2 cloves garlic, minced

- ¼ cup soy sauce
- 2 tablespoons oyster sauce
- 1 tablespoon cornstarch
- Salt and pepper to taste

Instructions:

1. In a big skillet or wok, heat the vegetable oil over high heat.

2. Put the garlic along with the beef, and allow to cook till the beef becomes brown.

3. Combine the cornstarch, oyster sauce, and soy sauce in a small mixing bowl and whisk. Stir well after adding the sauce to the beef.

4. When the broccoli florets are tender-crisp, put them inside the skillet and cook for a few minutes.

5. To get a taste, season the food with salt and pepper.For one more minute, stir-fry.

6. Serve hot alongside steamed rice or noodles.

Chicken and Vegetable Stir-Fry

Servings: 4

Cooking time: 25 minutes

Ingredients:

- One pound of sliced, skinless, boneless chicken breasts
- 2 tablespoons vegetable oil
- 2 cloves garlic, minced
- 1 red bell pepper, thinly sliced
- 1 green bell pepper, thinly sliced
- 1 small zucchini, sliced
- 1 cup broccoli florets
- ½ cup low-sodium soy sauce
- 2 tablespoons honey
- 1 tablespoon cornstarch
- Salt and pepper to taste

Instructions:

1. In a big skillet or wok, heat the vegetable oil over a high flame.

2. Cook until the chicken is browned after adding the chicken and the garlic.

3. Sliced broccoli, zucchini, and bell peppers should be added to the skillet.

4. Vegetables should be stir-fried for just a few minutes until crisp-tender.

5. Combine the soy sauce, honey, cornstarch, salt, and pepper in a small mixing bowl and whisk. Over the chicken and vegetables, pour the sauce.

6. Mix very well and cook for another extra minute till the sauce has thickened and coated the ingredients.

7. Serve hot alongside steamed rice or noodles.

Cheesy Baked Pasta

Servings: 6

Cooking time: 45 minutes

Ingredients:
- 12 ounces penne pasta
- 2 tablespoons butter
- 1 small onion, finely chopped
- 2 cloves garlic, minced

- 1 pound ground beef
- 1 can (14 ounces) diced tomatoes, drained
- 1 can (8 ounces) tomato sauce
- 1 teaspoon dried basil
- 1 teaspoon dried oregano
- ½ teaspoon salt
- ½ teaspoon black pepper
- 1 cup shredded mozzarella cheese
- ½ cup grated Parmesan cheese

Instructions:

1. Set the oven's temperature to 375°F (190°C).

2. The penne pasta should be prepared according to the instructions on the package. Drain, then set apart.

3. Melt the butter in a sizable skillet over a medium flame.

4. Sauté the onion and garlic after being added until they are aromatic and soft.

5. Brown the ground beef in the skillet after adding it. Remove any extra fat.

6. Add the tomato sauce, diced tomatoes, dried oregano, dried basil, salt, and black pepper. Then use five minutes to simmer it.

7. The cooked pasta and the beef mixture should be combined in a sizable baking dish. To coat the pasta, thoroughly mix.

8. Top with grated Parmesan cheese and mozzarella cheese that has been shredded.

9. Bake for twenty to twenty-five minutes in a preheated oven, till the cheese becomes melted and bubbly.

10. Enjoy and serve while hot.

Salmon with Roasted Vegetables

Servings: 4

Cooking time: 30 minutes

Ingredients:
- 4 salmon fillets
- 2 tablespoons olive oil
- 1 teaspoon dried dill
- ½ teaspoon garlic powder

- ½ teaspoon paprika
- Salt and pepper to taste
- 2 cups broccoli florets
- 2 cups cauliflower florets
- 1 red bell pepper, sliced
- 1 yellow bell pepper, sliced
- 1 tablespoon balsamic vinegar

Instructions:

1. Set the oven's temperature to 400°F (200°C).

2. You should use parchment paper for covering a baking sheet.

3. Combine olive oil, paprika, dried dill, garlic powder, salt, and pepper in a small mixing container.

4. The salmon fillets should be rubbed and covered in the mixture.

5. On one side of the baking sheet that has been prepared, set up the salmon fillets.

6. Combine and mix the broccoli, cauliflower, red, and yellow bell pepper bites with the balsamic vinegar, olive oil, salt, and pepper in a separate bowl.

7. On the opposite side of the baking sheet, distribute the vegetables.

8. The vegetables should be tender and the salmon should be cooked through after 20 minutes in the preheated oven.

9. Give it time to cool down after you bring it from the oven.

10. Serve the roasted salmon alongside the vegetables.

Creamy Mushroom and Spinach Pasta

Servings: 4

Cooking time: 30 minutes

Ingredients:
- 12 ounces pasta (your choice)
- 2 tablespoons butter
- 8 ounces mushrooms, sliced
- 2 cloves garlic, minced
- 2 cups fresh spinach leaves

- 1 cup heavy cream
- ½ cup grated Parmesan cheese
- Salt and pepper to taste

Instructions:

1. As directed on the packaging, cook the pasta. Drain, then set apart.

2. Melt the butter in a sizable skillet over a medium flame.

3. Sauté the mushrooms until they are golden brown after adding the garlic.

4. To the skillet, add the spinach leaves, and stir frequently until wilted.

5. Add the heavy cream, then simmer the mixture.

6. As the sauce thickens, stir in the grated Parmesan cheese until it melts.

7. To get a taste, season the food with salt and pepper.

8. Pasta that has been cooked should be thoroughly coated in sauce.

9. Enjoy and serve while hot.

Loaded Sweet Potato Nachos

Servings: 4

Cooking time: 30 minutes

Ingredients:

- 4 large sweet potatoes, thinly sliced
- 2 tablespoons olive oil
- 1 teaspoon chilli powder
- 1 teaspoon paprika
- 1 teaspoon garlic powder
- 1 cup shredded cheddar cheese
- 1 cup cooked black beans
- 1 cup diced tomatoes
- 1/2 cup sliced black olives
- 1/4 cup sliced green onions
- Sour cream and guacamole (optional)
- Salt and pepper to taste

Instructions:

1. Set the oven's temperature to 425°F (220°C). You should use parchment paper for covering a baking sheet.

1. Slices of sweet potato should be mixed with olive oil, chilli powder, paprika, garlic powder, salt, and pepper in a big mixing bowl.

2. Place the seasoned sweet potato slices in a single layer on the baking sheet that has been prepared.

3. Bake the sweet potatoes in the preheated oven for 20 to 25 minutes, or until they are crispy and golden brown.

4. After taking the sweet potatoes out of the oven, evenly distribute the shredded cheddar cheese on top.

5. Add green onions, black beans, diced tomatoes, and black olives to the top.

6. To melt the cheese, put the dish back in the oven for an additional five minutes.

7. If desired, serve the loaded sweet potato nachos with guacamole and sour cream.

Shrimp and Avocado Salad

Servings: 2

Preparation time: 15 minutes

Ingredients:

- 1 pound cooked shrimp, peeled and deveined
- 1 avocado, diced
- 1 cup cherry tomatoes, halved
- 1/4 cup diced red onion
- 2 tablespoons chopped fresh cilantro
- Juice of 1 lime
- 1 tablespoon olive oil
- Salt and pepper to taste

Instructions:

1. The cooked shrimp, diced avocado, cherry tomatoes, red onion, and chopped cilantro should all be combined in a big bowl.

2. Olive oil, lime juice, salt, and pepper should all be combined and mixed in a small mixing bowl.

3. Over the shrimp and avocado mixture, drizzle the dressing.

4. Gently combine by tossing.

5. Serve the shrimp and avocado salad as a light and healthy alternative to dinner.

Beef and Barley Soup

Servings: 6

Cooking time: 1 hour 30 minutes

Ingredients:

- 1 pound beef stew meat, cubed
- 2 tablespoons vegetable oil
- 1 onion, chopped
- 2 carrots, chopped
- 2 celery stalks, chopped
- 2 cloves garlic, minced
- 6 cups beef broth
- 1 cup pearl barley
- 1 bay leaf
- 1 teaspoon dried thyme
- Salt and pepper to taste
- Chopped fresh parsley for garnish

Instructions:

1. Over medium heat, warm up the vegetable oil in a big pot or Dutch oven. Brown the beef stew meat completely before adding more.

2. Put the beef to one side, after removing it from the pot.

3. Add the chopped celery, onion, carrots, and garlic to the same pot.

4. The vegetables should be sautéed for a few minutes until tender.

5. Browned beef should be added back to the pot. Add the pearl barley, bay leaf, dried thyme, salt, and pepper along with the beef broth.

6. Reduce the heat after the soup comes to a boil.

7. Once the barley is cooked and the beef is tender, cover and simmer for about an hour.

8. From the soup, remove the bay leaf. If needed, adjust the seasoning.

Hot beef and barley soup should be served with fresh parsley that has been chopped.

Vegetarian Chickpea Curry

Servings: 4

Cooking time: 30 minutes

Ingredients:

- 2 tablespoons vegetable oil
- 1 onion, chopped
- 2 cloves garlic, minced
- 1 tablespoon grated ginger
- 2 teaspoons curry powder
- 1 teaspoon ground cumin
- 1/2 teaspoon ground turmeric
- 1/4 teaspoon cayenne pepper (optional)
- 1 can (14 ounces) diced tomatoes
- 1 can (14 ounces) of coconut milk
- Two cans of cleaned and drained chickpeas
- Salt and pepper to taste
- Chopped fresh cilantro for garnish

Instructions:

1. In a sizable skillet or pot set over medium heat, warm up the vegetable oil.

2. The chopped onion should be added and sautéed until translucent.

3. Garlic powder, ginger powder, cumin powder, turmeric powder, and cayenne pepper (if used) should all be added. Cook until aromatic for one more minute.

4. Add coconut milk and diced tomatoes after stirring. The mixture should be cooked briefly.

5. Put the chickpeas that have been cleaned and drained into the skillet.

6. To allow the flavours to meld, simmer for about 15 minutes

7. To taste, add salt and pepper to the food. If necessary, alter the spice blend.

8. With naan bread or over steaming rice, serve the vegetarian chickpea curry. As a garnish, include freshly chopped cilantro.

CHAPTER 5

SNACKS RECIPES

Trail Mix Energy Balls

Servings: 12

Cooking Time: 15 minutes

Ingredients:

- 1 cup rolled oats
- Half a cup of nut butter, like almond or peanut butter
- 1/4 cup honey or maple syrup
- 1/4 cup chopped nuts (e.g., almonds, walnuts)
- 1/4 cup dried fruit (e.g., raisins, cranberries)
- 1/4 cup mini chocolate chips
- 1 tablespoon chia seeds (optional)
- 1 teaspoon vanilla extract

Instructions:

1. In a mixing container, mix all the ingredients.

2. Stir thoroughly until the mixture is thoroughly blended.

3. Make balls out of the mixture by taking small amounts.

4. On a baking sheet with parchment paper, arrange the balls.

5. To firm up, refrigerate for about 30 minutes.

6. Transfer the energy balls to an airtight container once they are firm.

7. Eat as a snack and keep it in the refrigerator.

Nutella Banana Wrap

Servings: 1

Cooking Time: 5 minutes

Ingredients:
- 1 large tortilla or wrap
- 2 tablespoons Nutella
- 1 ripe banana
- Optional toppings: crushed nuts, shredded coconut

Instructions:
1. Place the wrap or tortilla on a neat surface.

2. Over the entire surface, evenly distribute the Nutella.

3. At one end of the tortilla, place a ripe banana, and tightly roll the tortilla up.

4. For optional flavour and texture, top with chopped nuts or shredded coconut.

5. Eat the wrap whole or cut it into bite-sized pieces.

6. Serve and enjoy the banana wrap with Nutella.

Banana Nut Muffins

Servings: 12

Cooking Time: 25 minutes

Ingredients:

- 2 ripe bananas, mashed
- 1/2 cup sugar
- 1/4 cup melted butter
- 1/4 cup milk
- 2 eggs
- 1 3/4 cups all-purpose flour
- 1 teaspoon baking powder
- 1/2 teaspoon baking soda
- 1/4 teaspoon salt
- 1/2 cup chopped nuts (e.g., walnuts, pecans)

Instructions:

1. Set the oven's temperature to 375°F (190°C). Lubricate or line a muffin tin.

2. The mashed bananas, sugar, melted butter, milk, and eggs should all be combined in a mixing container.

3. Mix the flour, baking soda, baking powder, and salt in a different bowl.

4. Stirring to just combine, gradually add the dry ingredients to the banana mixture.

5. Add the chopped nuts and stir.

6. By evenly dividing the batter among the muffin tins and filling each one about 3/4 full.

7. A toothpick inserted into the centre of a muffin should come out clean after twenty to twenty-five minutes of baking.

8. After removing from the oven, let the muffins cool in the pan for a short while.

9. Place the muffins on a wire rack to finish cooling.

10. Serve and enjoy the banana nut muffins as a tasty snack.

Loaded Nachos

Servings: 2

Cooking Time: 15 minutes

Ingredients:
- 1 bag tortilla chips
- A single cup of cooked ground beef or sliced chicken
- A cup of grated cheese, such as cheddar or Monterey jack
- 1/4 cup diced tomatoes
- 1/4 cup diced bell peppers
- 1/4 cup sliced black olives
- 1/4 cup chopped green onions
- Optional toppings: sour cream, guacamole, salsa

Instructions:
1. Set the oven's temperature to 350°F (175°C).

2. On a baking sheet, spread the tortilla chips out.

3. Over the chips, evenly distribute the cooked ground beef or chicken shredded.

4. On top of the meat, strew the grated cheese.

5. Put the green onions, black olives, bell peppers, and diced tomatoes.

6. For about ten minutes, bake in the oven, or until the cheese is melted.

7. Take it out of the oven, then allow it to cool a little.

8. If desired, serve the loaded nachos alongside salsa, guacamole, or sour cream.

Chocolate Protein Balls

Servings: 12

Cooking Time: 15 minutes

Ingredients:
- 1 cup rolled oats
- 1/2 cup chocolate protein powder
- 1/4 cup almond butter or peanut butter

- 1/4 cup honey or maple syrup
- 1/4 cup mini chocolate chips
- 1 teaspoon vanilla extract
- Optional coatings: shredded coconut, cocoa powder, crushed nuts

Instructions:

1. Rolling oats, chocolate protein powder, almond butter, honey, mini chocolate chips, and vanilla extract should all be combined in a mixing container.

2. Stir thoroughly until the mixture is thoroughly blended.

3. Make balls out of the mixture by taking small amounts.

4. To give the balls different coatings, you could optionally roll them in chopped nuts, cocoa powder, or shredded coconut.

5. On a baking sheet with parchment paper, arrange the balls.

6. To firm up, refrigerate for about thirty minutes.

7. Transfer the protein balls to an airtight container once they are firm.

8. Enjoy as a protein-rich snack after storing it in the refrigerator.

CHAPTER 6

DESSERT RECIPES

Rice Pudding

Servings: 4

Cooking Time: 40 minutes

Ingredients:

- ½ cup uncooked white rice
- 4 cups whole milk
- ½ cup sugar
- 1 teaspoon vanilla extract
- Ground cinnamon for sprinkling

Instructions:

1. Drain the rice after giving it a cold water rinse.

2. Rice, milk, and sugar should be combined in a pan.

3. Cook for thirty to thirty-five stirring frequently, over a medium flame, or until the rice is tender and the mixture thickens.

4. After removing the pan from the heat, pour the vanilla extract.

5. To serve, divide the rice pudding among bowls and top with ground cinnamon.

6. Serve warm or cold.

Avocado Chocolate Mousse

Servings: 2

Cooking Time: 10 minutes

Ingredients:
- 2 ripe avocados
- ¼ cup cocoa powder
- ¼ cup honey or maple syrup
- ½ teaspoon vanilla extract
- Pinch of salt
- Optional toppings: whipped cream, berries, or shaved chocolate

Instructions:

1. The avocado flesh should be removed and put in a food processor or blender.

2. Salt, vanilla extract, honey or maple syrup, cocoa powder, and cocoa powder should be added.

3. Blend until it's creamy and smooth, scraping the sides as necessary.

4. Arrange the mousse serving bowls in the fridge for at least one hour.

5. Prior to serving, top with whipped cream, berries, or shaved chocolate.

Apple Crumble

Servings: 6

Cooking Time: 45 minutes

Ingredients:

- 4 medium-sized apples, peeled, cored, and sliced
- 1 tablespoon lemon juice
- ¼ cup granulated sugar

- ½ teaspoon ground cinnamon
- ½ cup all-purpose flour
- ½ cup rolled oats
- ½ cup brown sugar
- ¼ teaspoon salt
- 6 tablespoons unsalted butter, cold and cubed

Instructions:

1. Set the oven's temperature to 375°F (190°C).

2. Slices of apple should be coated with cinnamon, sugar, and lemon juice in a bowl.

3. In a baking pan, place the apple mixture.

4. The flour, rolled oats, brown sugar, and salt should all be combined in a separate bowl.

5. When the mixture resembles coarse crumbs, add the cold cubed butter and work it into the dry ingredients with your fingers or a pastry cutter.

6. Over the apples, distribute the crumb mixture evenly.

7. Bake for 30 to 35 minutes or till the topping is golden brown and the apples are tender.

8. Before serving, let it cool a little.

Chocolate Chip Cookie Bars

Servings: 12

Cooking Time: 25 minutes

Ingredients:

- 2 ¼ cups all-purpose flour
- 1 teaspoon baking soda
- ½ teaspoon salt
- 1 cup unsalted butter, softened
- ¾ cup granulated sugar
- ¾ cup brown sugar
- 2 large eggs
- 1 teaspoon vanilla extract
- 2 cups chocolate chips
- Optional: chopped nuts or additional toppings

Instructions:

1. Lubricate a 9x13-inch baking pan and set the oven to 350°F (175°C).

2. Mix and whisk the flour, baking soda, and salt in a medium bowl.

3. Softened butter, granulated sugar, and brown sugar should be creamed until light and fluffy in a large mixing bowl.

4. One at a time, beat in each egg, then add the vanilla extract.

5. After incorporating the dry ingredients into the wet ones gradually, mix just until combined.

6. Add the chocolate chips and, if desired, the chopped nuts.

7. In the prepared baking pan, evenly distribute the cookie dough.

8. Bake for twenty to twenty-five minutes till the edges are golden brown and a toothpick inserted into the middle comes out with a few moist crumbs.

9. Before cutting the cookie bars into squares, let them cool down completely.

Strawberry Cheesecake Bites

Servings: 12

Cooking Time: 30 minutes (plus chilling time)

Ingredients:

- 1 ½ cups graham cracker crumbs
- ¼ cup melted butter
- 1 cup cream cheese, softened
- ¼ cup powdered sugar
- 1 teaspoon vanilla extract
- Fresh strawberries, halved
- Strawberry sauce or jam for topping

Instructions:

1. Graham cracker crumbs and melted butter should be thoroughly mixed in a bowl.

2. To create a crust, press the mixture firmly into the bottom of a greased 9x9-inch baking dish.

3. Beat the cream cheese, powdered sugar, and vanilla extract until they are smooth and creamy in a different bowl.

4. Evenly distribute the cream cheese mixture over the crust.

5. The cream cheese layer should be followed by the strawberry halves.

6. Over the strawberries, apply a thin layer of strawberry jam or strawberry sauce.

7. To allow the flavours to meld and the cheesecake to set, place in the refrigerator for at least two hours.

8. Before serving, divide into bite-sized squares.

CHAPTER 7

SMOOTHIE RECIPES

Banana Peanut Butter Smoothie

Servings: 1

Cooking Time: 5 minutes

Ingredients:

- 1 ripe banana
- 2 tablespoons peanut butter
- 1 cup whole milk
- 1 tablespoon honey
- 1/2 teaspoon vanilla extract
- Ice cubes (optional)

Instructions:

1. Put the banana in the blender after peeling it.

2. Add ice cubes (if desired), whole milk, honey, vanilla extract, and peanut butter.

3. Blend till it becomes creamy and smooth.

4. Pour into a glass, then sip.

Chocolate Avocado Protein Smoothie

Servings: 1

Cooking Time: 5 minutes

Ingredients:

- 1/2 ripe avocado
- 1 cup almond milk
- 1 scoop of chocolate protein powder
- 1 tablespoon cocoa powder
- 1 tablespoon honey or maple syrup
- Ice cubes (optional)

Instructions:

1. Avocado flesh should be removed and put in a blender.

2. Add the following ingredients: cocoa powder, chocolate protein powder, honey, maple syrup, and ice cubes if you wish.

3. Blend till it becomes creamy and smooth.

4. Pour into a glass, then sip.

Berry Oatmeal Smoothie

Servings: 1

Cooking Time: 10 minutes

Ingredients:

- 1/2 cup rolled oats
- 1 cup mixed berries (strawberries, blueberries, raspberries)
- 1 cup milk or yoghurt
- 1 tablespoon honey or agave syrup
- 1/2 teaspoon vanilla extract
- Ice cubes (optional)

Instructions:

1. Rolled oats should be added to a blender and processed into a powder.

2. Ice cubes (if you like), milk, yoghurt, honey, agave syrup, vanilla extract, and mixed berries should all be added.

3. Blend till it becomes creamy and smooth.

4. Pour into a glass, then sip.

Peanut Butter and Jelly Smoothie

Servings: 1

Cooking Time: 5 minutes

Ingredients:

- 1 cup frozen mixed berries
- 2 tablespoons peanut butter
- 1 cup almond milk
- 1 tablespoon honey or agave syrup
- Ice cubes (optional)

Instructions:

1. Add a mixture of frozen berries in a blender.

2. Add ice cubes(if you like), honey or agave syrup, almond milk, and peanut butter.

3. Blend till it becomes creamy and smooth.

4. Pour into a glass, then sip.

Vanilla Berry Protein Smoothie

Servings: 1

Cooking Time: 5 minutes

Ingredients:

- 1 cup mixed berries (strawberries, blueberries, raspberries)
- 1 scoop vanilla protein powder
- 1 cup almond milk
- 1 tablespoon honey or agave syrup
- Ice cubes (optional)

Instructions:

1. Put a mixture of berries in a blender.

2. Add ice cubes (if you like), vanilla protein powder, almond milk, honey, or agave syrup.

3. Blend till smooth and creamy in consistency.

4. Pour into a glass, then sip.

Spinach and Mango Smoothie

Servings: 1

Cooking Time: 5 minutes

Ingredients:

- 1 cup fresh spinach leaves
- 1 ripe mango, peeled and pitted
- 1/2 cup Greek yoghurt
- 1 tablespoon honey or maple syrup
- Ice cubes (optional)

Instructions:

1. In a blender, add fresh spinach leaves.

2. Add Greek yoghurt, honey or maple syrup, ripe mango, and ice cubes (if you like).

3. Blend till smooth and creamy in consistency.

4. Pour into a glass, then sip.

Coconut Banana Almond Smoothie

Servings: 1

Cooking Time: 5 minutes

Ingredients:

- 1 ripe banana
- 1/4 cup almond butter
- 1 cup coconut milk
- 1 tablespoon honey or agave syrup
- Ice cubes (optional)

Instructions:

1. Put the banana in the blender after peeling it.

2. Add ice cubes (if you like), honey or agave syrup, coconut milk, and almond butter.

3. Blend till smooth and creamy in consistency.

4. Pour into a glass, then sip.

Cherry Almond Smoothie

Servings: 1

Cooking Time: 5 minutes

Ingredients:

- 1 cup frozen cherries
- 1/4 cup almond butter
- 1 cup almond milk
- 1 tablespoon honey or agave syrup
- Ice cubes (optional)

Instructions:

1. Put frozen cherries in a food processor or blender.

2. Add ice cubes(if you like), honey or agave syrup, almond milk, and almond butter.

3. Blend till smooth and creamy in consistency.

4. Pour into a glass, then sip.

Vanilla Almond Protein Smoothie

Servings: 1

Cooking Time: 5 minutes

Ingredients:

- 1 cup almond milk
- 1 scoop vanilla protein powder
- 1/4 cup almond butter
- 1 tablespoon honey or agave syrup
- Ice cubes (optional)

Instructions:

1. Put almond milk in a food processor or blender.

2. Add ice cubes (if you like), almond butter, honey or agave syrup, and vanilla protein powder.

3. Blend till smooth and creamy in consistency.

4. Pour into a glass, then sip.

Mango Banana Coconut Chia Smoothie

Servings: 1

Cooking Time: 5 minutes

Ingredients:

- 1 ripe mango, peeled and pitted
- 1 ripe banana
- 1/2 cup coconut milk
- 1 tablespoon chia seeds
- 1 tablespoon honey or maple syrup
- Ice cubes (optional)

Instructions:

1. Cut and place the chunks of the ripe mango in the blender.

2. Add ice cubes (if you like), a ripe banana, coconut milk, chia seeds, honey, or maple syrup.

3. Blend till smooth and creamy in consistency.

4. Pour into a glass, then sip.

CHAPTER 8

Tips and Tricks for Successful Weight Gain

Tracking Progress And Adjusting The Diet

Gaining weight can be just as difficult as losing it, so it's important to take a calculated approach to ensure healthy and long-lasting results. A successful weight gain journey must include tracking your progress and modifying your diet. Here are some pointers and techniques to help you efficiently monitor your development and make the necessary dietary changes:

1. **Set Clear Specific Goals:** Begin by establishing specific, attainable goals for weight gain. Decide how much weight you want to gain and when you want to do it. You'll have a benchmark to compare your advancement to thanks to this.

2. **Keep an Eye on Your Weight:** Weigh yourself frequently, ideally every week at the same time and day. Record your weight measurements so you can monitor any changes over time. Keep in mind that you should aim to gain 0.5 to 1 pound of weight per week, gradually and steadily.

3. **Track Body Measurements:** In addition to keeping an eye on your weight, you should also keep track of your hip, waist, and body fat percentage measurements. This will enable you to evaluate your overall progress and adjustments to your body's composition.

4. **Keep a Food Journal:** Keep a thorough food journal to keep tabs on your daily caloric intake. Take note of everything you eat and drink, along with the serving sizes and preparation techniques. To find out the nutritional value of your meals, use online databases or calorie-tracking apps.

5. **Calculate Caloric Needs:** To estimate how many calories you need each day to gain weight, use an online calorie counter or speak with a registered dietitian. To support gradual weight gain, try to eat more calories than you need—typically 250–500 more than what you need for maintenance.

6. **Focus on Nutrient-Dense Foods:** Choose foods high in vitamins, minerals, complex carbohydrates, healthy fats, and lean proteins that are nutrient-dense. Include a variety

of sources in your diet, such as lean meats, fish, poultry, whole grains, legumes, nuts, seeds, fruits, and vegetables.

7. **Increase Meal Frequency**: Try consuming your calories in five or six smaller meals and snacks throughout the day rather than three large meals a day. You may be able to more easily meet your caloric needs using this strategy.

8. **Keep an eye on Macronutrient Ratios:** Keep an eye on how your macronutrients are distributed. Prioritize a balanced intake of protein and good fats over carbohydrates, even though they are necessary for energy. Aim for 20–30% of calories coming from protein, 20–35% from fats, and the rest from carbohydrates.

9. **Regularly Evaluate Progress:** Every two to four weeks, evaluate how much weight you have gained. To gauge your progress, review your food diary, body measurements, and weight fluctuations. Consider modifying your caloric intake if you're not gaining weight at the desired rate.

10. **Seek Expert Advice:** Speaking with a registered dietitian or nutritionist who focuses on weight gain can offer individualized advice and support. They can provide

recommendations for calorie-dense foods, assist you in creating a customized meal plan, and address any nutritional issues.

11. **Be Patient and Consistent:** Keep in mind that weight gain and loss both require patience. Be persistent and patient in your efforts. Give your body time to adapt and grow by gradually changing your diet and way of life.

12. **Stay Active:** Perform regular resistance training exercises to help build muscle and prevent gaining too much fat. Maintain your overall fitness by combining strength training with cardiovascular exercise to help you gain weight.

It's important to find a strategy that works best for you because every person's body is different. You can achieve your weight gain objectives healthily and sustainably by monitoring your progress and modifying your diet as a result of the feedback you receive.

Incorporating Exercise And Strength Training

It takes a combination of good nutrition and exercise to gain weight in a healthy and controlled way. While a lot of people concentrate on losing weight, some people aim to gain weight for a variety of reasons, such as gaining muscle mass, healing from an illness, or just improving their body composition in general. Achieving your weight gain objectives can be greatly aided by incorporating exercise and strength training into your routine. Following are some pointers and techniques for successfully gaining weight through exercise:

1. **Set Realistic Timelines and Specific Goals:** Specify your objectives for weight gain. You'll be more focused and motivated throughout your journey if you have a clear target weight and time frame.

2. **Consult A Professional:** A qualified fitness professional, such as a personal trainer or a registered dietitian, should be consulted before beginning any exercise or strength training program. They can help you create a custom plan based on your present level of fitness, body type, and requirements.

3. **Concentrate on Compound Exercises:** Include compound exercises in your routine because they work for multiple muscle groups at once. Squats, dead lifts, bench presses, and overhead presses are all great exercises for promoting muscle growth and boosting overall strength.

4. **Progressive Overload:** By incorporating the concept of progressive overload, you can gradually raise the intensity of your workouts. To consistently challenge your muscles and promote growth, this entails gradually increasing the weight, repetitions, or sets.

5. **Strength Training Frequency:** Aim to strength train at least twice or three times a week, with enough time in between to recover. While preventing overtraining, this frequency will give your muscles the stimulus they need to grow.

6. **Maximize Your Workout Volume:** To gain weight, you must perform a sufficient number of exercises. This is possible by performing several sets (about 3) of each exercise, with a high to moderate number of repetitions (8–12) per set.

7. **Include Caloric Surplus:** Make sure you are consuming an excess of calories to support weight gain. To encourage gradual weight gain, determine your daily caloric needs and add an extra 250–500 calories per day. Lean proteins, whole grains, fruits, vegetables, and healthy fats are foods that are high in nutrients.

8. **Sufficient Protein Intake:** A sufficient protein intake is essential for muscle growth and repair. 1.2–1.6 grams of protein per kilogram of body weight should be consumed each day. Include plant-based protein sources in your diet along with lean meats, fish, eggs, dairy, and legumes.

9. **Optimal Rest and Recovery:** The best rest and recovery are achieved by giving your body adequate downtime in between workouts. For muscles to repair and grow, you must get enough sleep, control your stress levels, and schedule rest days into your training schedule.

10. **Monitor and Modify:** Keep tabs on your development and alter your diet and exercise schedule as necessary. If you're not getting the desired results, seek professional advice to adjust your strategy.

Keep in mind that healthy weight gain requires patience and consistency. Maintain a consistent exercise and strength training schedule, feed your body the proper nutrients, and exercise patience as the process unfolds. You can achieve your weight gain objectives and enhance your general health and fitness with commitment and perseverance.

CONCLUSION

The Weight Gain Diet Cookbook For Beginners is not just a book, it is a comprehensive guide that provides readers with the tools they need to transform their bodies and lives. With its easy-to-follow recipes and practical tips, this book is a must-read for anyone who wants to gain weight healthily and sustainably.

By following the advice and guidance provided in this book, you have the power to transform your body, boost your confidence, and live your best life. As a beginner , this book is sure to become your go-to guide for healthy weight gain. With its wealth of information and delicious recipes, the Weight Gain Diet Cookbook For Beginners is a must-have for anyone looking to take control of their health and achieve their weight gain goals.

Thank you for taking the time to read the Weight Gain Diet Cookbook For Beginners. We hope that this book has provided you with the knowledge and tools you need to achieve your weight gain goals healthily and sustainably. Remember, taking care of your health is a journey, and we are honoured to be a part of yours. So go ahead and start cooking those delicious recipes and enjoy the benefits of a balanced diet. Thank you again for choosing our book, and we wish you all the best on your health journey!

BONUS

21 Days Meal Plan

Day 1

Breakfast: Protein Pancakes with Toppings

Lunch: Protein-Packed Lentil Salad

Dinner: Loaded Sweet Potato Nachos

Day 2

Breakfast: Oatmeal Power Bowl

Lunch: Salmon and Quinoa Salad

Dinner: Shrimp and Avocado Salad

Day 3

Breakfast: Banana Nut Overnight Oat

Lunch: Loaded Chicken Salad Sandwich

Dinner: Beef and Barley Soup

Day 4

Breakfast: High-Calorie Smoothie Bowl

Lunch: Cheesy Baked Potatoes

Dinner: Creamy Mushroom and Spinach Pasta

Day 5

Breakfast: Energy-Packed Breakfast Burrito

Lunch: Loaded Turkey Wrap

Dinner: Salmon With Roasted Vegetables

Day 6

Breakfast: Avocado and Egg Toast

Lunch: Tuna and Avocado Wrap

Dinner: Cheesy Baked Pasta

Day 7

Breakfast: High-Calorie Oatmeal

Lunch: Creamy Chicken Pasta

Dinner: Chicken and Vegetable Stir-Fry

Day 8

Breakfast: Chia Pudding with Berries

Lunch: Beef and Vegetable Stir-Fry

Dinner: Creamy Chicken Alfredo

Day 9

Breakfast: Veggie Breakfast Scramble

Lunch: Loaded Sweet Potato

Dinner: Beef and Broccoli Stir-Fry

Day 10

Breakfast: Sweet Potato Hash with Eggs

Lunch: Chickpea and Spinach Curry

Dinner: Vegetarian Chickpea Curry

Day 11

Breakfast: Energy-Packed Breakfast Burrito

Lunch: Salmon and Quinoa Salad

Dinner: Beef and Barley Soup

Day 12

Breakfast: Avocado and Egg Toast

Lunch: Loaded Chicken Salad Sandwich

Dinner: Creamy Mushroom and Spinach Pasta

Day 13

Breakfast: High-Calorie Oatmeal

Lunch: Cheesy Baked Potatoes

Dinner: Salmon With Roasted Vegetables

Day 14

Breakfast: Banana Nut Overnight Oat

Lunch: Beef and Vegetable Stir-Fry

Dinner: Vegetarian Chickpea Curry

Day 15

Breakfast: Oatmeal Power Bowl

Lunch: Loaded Sweet Potato

Dinner: Beef and Broccoli Stir-Fry

Day 16

Breakfast: Protein Pancakes With Toppings

Lunch: Chickpea and Spinach Curry

Dinner: Salmon With Roasted Vegetables

Day 17

Breakfast: Banana Nut Overnight Oat

Lunch: Protein-Packed Lentil Salad

Dinner: Creamy Chicken Alfredo

Day 18

Breakfast: Veggie Breakfast Scramble

Lunch: Loaded Turkey Wrap

Dinner: Cheesy Baked Pasta

Day 19

Breakfast: Sweet Potato Hash with Eggs

Lunch: Tuna and Avocado Wrap

Dinner: Chicken and Vegetable Stir-Fry

Day 20

Breakfast: Chia Pudding with Berries

Lunch: Creamy Chicken Pasta

Dinner: Loaded Sweet Potato Nachos

Day 21

Breakfast: Avocado and Egg Toast

Lunch: Salmon and Quinoa Salad

Dinner: Vegetarian Chickpea Curry